CW00450132

Lean and Green Plan in 50 Recipes

A Different Meal Every Day with This New
Cookbook

Carmen Bellisario

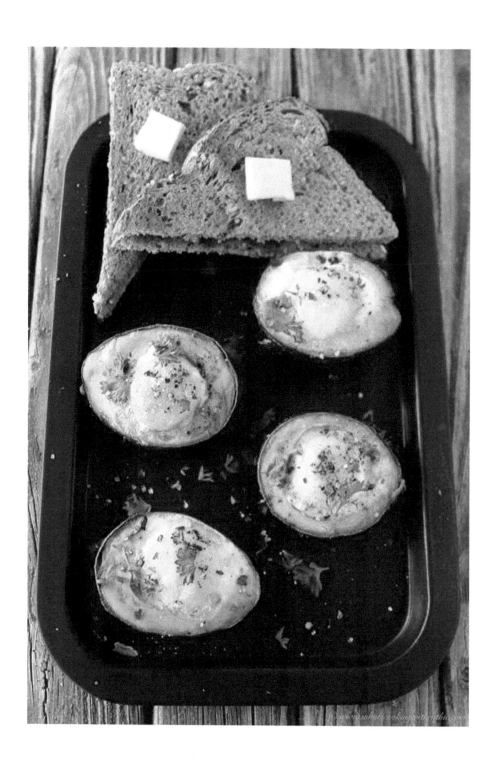

TABLE OF CONTENTS

CHICKEN & BELL PEPPER OMELET 7

TURKEY & ZUCCHINI OMELET 9

SPINACH & TOFU OMELET 11

MINI VEGGIE FRITTATAS 13

SPINACH & TOMATO FRITTATA 15

CHICKEN & VEGGIES FRITTATA 17

BEEF & SCALLION FRITTATA 19

BEEF & VEGGIE FRITTATA 21

PORK & SPINACH FRITTATA 23

TROUT FRITTATA 25

TOMATO QUICHE 27

SPINACH QUICHE 29

CHICKEN & SPINACH QUICHE 31

GROUND CHICKEN & MUSHROOM FRITTATA 33

SALMON QUICHE 35

BEEF & MUSHROOM CASSEROLE 37

CHICKEN & CAULIFLOWER CASSEROLE 39

EGGS WITH TURKEY & SPINACH 41

EGGS WITH TURKEY 43

CRANBERRY MUFFINS 45

SAVORY CARROT MUFFINS 47

CHICKEN & SPINACH MUFFINS...50

ZUCCHINI FRITTERS...52

ONION SOUP 54

MIXED VEGGIES SOUP 57

LEAN AND GREEN PIZZA HACK 59

AMARANTH PORRIDGE...61

LAVENDER BLUEBERRY CHIA SEED PUDDING 63

COCONUT CHIA PUDDING WITH BERRIES 65

OMELETTE WITH TOMATOES AND SPRING ONIONS 67

BACON CHEESEBURGER 69

CHIA SEED GEL WITH POMEGRANATE AND NUTS 71

PANCAKES WITH BERRIES 73

PORRIDGE WITH WALNUTS 75

OMELETTE À LA MARGHERITA..77

SWEET CASHEW CHEESE SPREAD...79

PERSONAL BISCUIT PIZZA 81

FRIED EGG WITH BACON...83

EEL ON SCRAMBLED EGGS AND BREAD..84

WHOLE GRAIN BREAD AND AVOCADO 86

CHEESEBURGER PIE...88

ASPARAGUS & CRABMEAT FRITTATA 90

GRILLED CHICKEN POWER BOWL WITH GREEN GODDESS DRESSING 92

YOGURT WITH GRANOLA AND PERSIMMON 94

SMOOTHIE BOWL WITH SPINACH, MANGO, AND MUESLI....................................96

SMOOTHIE BOWL WITH BERRIES, POPPY SEEDS, NUTS AND SEEDS......................98

MINI ZUCCHINI BITES...100

BEEF WITH BROCCOLI ON CAULIFLOWER RICE...102

ANCHO TILAPIA ON CAULIFLOWER RICE 104

TURKEY CAPRESE MEATLOAF CUPS 106

ALMOND PANCAKES..108

Chicken & Bell Pepper Omelet

Servings: 5

Preparation time: 15 minutes

Cooking time: 2¾ minutes

Ingredients:

- ½ cup of unsweetened almond milk
- 6 eggs
- 1 garlic clove, minced
- Salt and ground black pepper, as required
- ¾ cup of cooked chicken, chopped
- 1 red bell pepper, seeded and sliced thinly
- 1 small white onion, chopped finely
- 1 cup of part-skim mozzarella cheese, shredded

Instructions:

1. In a bowl, add the milk, eggs, garlic, salt and black pepper and beat until well combined.
2. In a greased baking dish, place the egg mixture.
3. Add the chicken, bell pepper and onion and stir to mix.
4. Arrange the baking dish over the wire rack.

5. Select "Slow Cooker" of Breville Smart Air Fryer Oven and assail "High".

6. Set the timer for 2¾ hours and press "Start/Stop" to start cooking.

7. After 2½ hours, sprinkle the omelets with cheese evenly.

8. When the Cooking time is completed, remove the baking dish from the oven and transfer the omelets onto a serving plate.

9. Cut into 4 equal-sized wedges and serve hot.

Turkey & Zucchini Omelet

Servings: 6

Preparation time: 15 minutes

Cooking time: 35 minutes

Ingredients:

- 8 eggs
- ½ cup of unsweetened almond milk
- 1/8 teaspoon of red pepper flakes, crushed
- Salt and ground black pepper, as required
- 1 cup of cooked turkey meat, chopped
- 1 cup of low-fat Monterrey Jack cheese, shredded
- ½ cup of fresh scallion, chopped
- ¾ cup of zucchini, chopped

Instructions:

1. In a bowl, add the eggs, almond milk, salt and black pepper and beat well.
2. Add the remaining Ingredients and stir to mix.
3. Place the mixture into a greased baking dish.

4. Select "Bake" of Breville Smart Air Fryer Oven and adjust the temperature to 315 degrees F.

5. Set the timer for 35 minutes and press "Start/Stop" to start preheating.

6. When the unit beeps to point out that it's preheated, arrange the baking dish over the wire rack.

7. When the Cooking time is completed, remove the baking dish from the oven and place onto a wire rack to chill for about 5 minutes before serving.

8. Cut into equal-sized wedges and serve.

Spinach & Tofu Omelet

Servings: 2

Preparation time: 15 minutes

Cooking time: 10 minutes

Ingredients:

- 1 teaspoon of arrowroot starch
- 2 teaspoons of water
- 3 eggs
- 2 teaspoons of red boat fish sauce
- 1 teaspoon of olive oil
- Ground black pepper, as required
- ¼ cup of fresh spinach, chopped finely
- 6 ounces of silken tofu, pressed and sliced

Instructions:

1. In a large bowl, dissolve arrowroot starch in water.
2. Add the eggs, fish sauce, oil and black pepper and beat well.
3. Add the spinach and stir to mix.

4. Place tofu in the bottom of a greased baking dish and top with the egg mixture.
5. Select "Air Fry" of Breville Smart Air Fryer Oven and adjust the temperature to 390 degrees F.
6. Set the timer for 10 minutes and press "Start/Stop" to start preheating.
7. When the unit beeps to point out that it's preheated, arrange the baking dish over the wire rack.
8. When the Cooking time is completed, remove the baking dish from oven and place onto a wire rack to chill for about 5 minutes before serving.
9. Cut into equal-sized wedges and serve.

Mini Veggie Frittatas

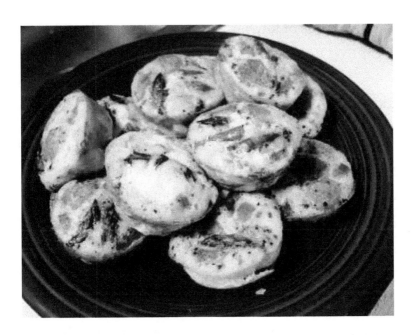

Servings: 2

Preparation time: 15 minutes

Cooking time: 17 minutes

Ingredients:

- 1 tablespoon of coconut oil
- ½ of white onion sliced thinly
- 1 cup of fresh mushrooms, sliced thinly
- 1¼ cups of fresh spinach, chopped
- 3 eggs

- ½ teaspoon of fresh rosemary, chopped
- Salt and ground black pepper, as required
- 3 tablespoons of low-fat Parmesan cheese, shredded

Instructions:

1. In a frying pan, melt coconut oil over medium heat and cook the onion and mushroom for about 3 minutes.
2. Add the spinach and cook for about 2-3 minutes.
3. Remove the frying pan from heat and put aside to chill slightly.
4. Meanwhile, in a small bowl, add the eggs, rosemary, salt and black pepper and beat well.
5. Divide the beaten eggs into 2 greased ramekins evenly and top with the veggie mixture, followed by the cheese.
6. Select "Air Fry" of Breville Smart Air Fryer Oven and adjust the temperature to 330 degrees F.
7. Set the timer for 12 minutes and press "Start/Stop" to start preheating.
8. When the unit beeps to point out that it's preheated, place the ramekins over the air rack.
9. When the Cooking time is completed, remove the ramekins from oven and place onto a wire rack for about 5 minutes before serving.

Spinach & Tomato Frittata

Servings: 6

Preparation time: 15 minutes

Cooking time: 30 minutes

Ingredients:

- 10 large eggs
- Salt and ground black pepper, as required
- 1 (5-ounce of) bag baby spinach
- 2 cups of grape tomatoes, halved
- 4 scallions, sliced thinly
- 8 ounces of feta cheese, crumbled
- 3 tablespoons of hot olive oil

Instructions:

1. In a bowl, place the eggs, salt and black pepper and beat well.
2. Add the spinach, tomatoes, scallions and feta cheese and gently stir to mix.
3. Spread the oil in a baking dish and top with the spinach mixture.

4. Select "Bake" of Breville Smart Air Fryer Oven and adjust the temperature to 350 degrees F.

5. Set the timer for 30 minutes and press "Start/Stop" to start preheating.

6. When the unit beeps to point out that it's preheated, arrange the baking dish over the wire rack.

7. When the Cooking time is completed, remove the baking dish from oven and place onto a wire rack to chill for about 5 minutes before serving.

8. Cut into equal-sized wedges and serve.

Chicken & Veggies Frittata

Servings: 8

Preparation time: 15 minutes

Cooking time: 3 hours

Ingredients:

- 8 eggs
- ½ teaspoon of dried parsley
- Pinch of garlic powder
- Salt and ground black pepper, as required
- 1 1/3 cups of cooked chicken, chopped finely
- 1½ cups of red bell pepper, seeded and chopped
- ¾ cup of frozen chopped spinach, thawed and squeezed
- ¼ cup of yellow onion, chopped

Instructions:

1. In a bowl, add the eggs, parsley, garlic powder, salt and black pepper and beat well.
2. In a greased baking dish, place the remaining Ingredients.

3. Pour the egg mixture over chicken mixture and gently stir to mix.

4. Arrange the baking dish over the wire rack.

5. Select "Slow Cooker" of Breville Smart Air Fryer Oven and assail "Low".

6. Set the timer for 3 hours and press "Start/Stop" to start cooking.

7. When the Cooking time is completed, remove the baking dish from the oven and transfer the frittata onto a serving plate.

8. Cut into 4 equal-sized wedges and serve hot.

Beef & Scallion Frittata

Servings: 4

Preparation time: 15 minutes

Cooking time: 20 minutes

Ingredients:

- ½ pound cooked ground beef, grease removed
- 1 cup of low-fat Colby Jack cheese, shredded
- 8 eggs, beaten lightly
- 4 scallions, chopped
- 1/8 teaspoon of red pepper flakes, crushed
- Salt and ground black pepper, as required

Instructions:

1. In a bowl, add the meat, cheese, eggs, scallion and cayenne and blend until well combined.
2. Place the mixture into a greased baking dish.
3. Select "Air Fry" of Breville Smart Air Fryer Oven and adjust the temperature to 360 degrees F.
4. Set the timer for 20 minutes and press "Start/Stop" to start preheating.

5. When the unit beeps to point out that it's preheated, arrange the baking dish over the wire rack.

6. When the Cooking time is completed, remove the baking dish from oven and place onto a wire rack to chill for about 5 minutes before serving.

7. Cut into 4 wedges and serve.

Beef & Veggie Frittata

Servings: 2

Preparation time: 15 minutes

Cooking time: 14 minutes

Ingredients:

- 1 tablespoon of olive oil
- ¼ cup of cooked ground beef
- 4 cherry tomatoes, halved
- 6 fresh mushrooms, sliced
- Salt and ground black pepper, as required
- 3 eggs
- 1 tablespoon of fresh parsley, chopped
- ½ cup of low-fat Parmesan cheese, grated

Instructions:

1. In a baking dish, place the bacon, tomatoes, mushrooms, salt, and black pepper and blend well.
2. Place the baking dish in the air fry basket.
3. Select "Air Fry" of Breville Smart Air Fryer Oven and adjust the temperature to 320 degrees F.

4. Set the timer for 14 minutes and press "Start/Stop" to start preheating.
5. When the unit beeps to point out that it's preheated, insert the air fry basket in the oven.
6. Meanwhile, in a bowl, add the eggs and beat well.
7. Add the parsley and cheese and blend well.
8. After 6 minutes of cooking, top the bacon mixture with egg mixture evenly.
9. When the Cooking time is completed, remove the air fry basket from the oven and transfer the frittata onto a plate.
10. Cut into equal-sized wedges and serve hot.

Pork & Spinach Frittata

Servings: 2

Preparation time: 15 minutes

Cooking time: 13 minutes

Ingredients:

- ¼ cup of cooked pork, chopped
- ½ tomato, cubed
- ¼ cup of fresh baby spinach
- 3 eggs
- Salt and ground black pepper, as required
- ¼ cup of low-fat Parmesan cheese, grated

Instructions:

1. In a skillet, heat the oil over medium heat, cook the pork and tomato and cook for about 5 minutes.
2. Add the spinach and cook for about 1-2 minutes.
3. Remove from the heat and put aside to chill slightly.
4. Meanwhile, in a small bowl, add the eggs, salt and black pepper and beat well.

5. In a baking dish, place the pork mixture and top with egg mixture.

6. Select "Air Fry" of Breville Smart Air Fryer Oven and adjust the temperature to 355 degrees F.

7. Set the timer for 8 minutes and press "Start/Stop" to start preheating.

8. When the unit beeps to point out that it's preheated, arrange the baking dish over the wire rack.

9. When the Cooking time is completed, remove the baking dish from oven and transfer the frittata onto a platter.

10. Cut into equal-sized wedges and serve hot.

Trout Frittata

Servings: 4

Preparation time: 15 minutes

Cooking time: 25 minutes

Ingredients:

- 1 tablespoon of olive oil
- 1 onion, sliced
- 6 eggs
- ½ tablespoon of horseradish sauce
- 2 tablespoons of crème Fraiche
- 2 hot-smoked trout fillets, chopped
- ¼ cup of fresh dill, chopped

Instructions:

1. In a skillet, heat the oil over medium heat and cook the onion for about 4-5 minutes.
2. Remove from the heat and put aside.
3. Meanwhile, in a bowl, add the eggs, sauce Albert, and crème Fraiche and blend well.

4. In the bottom of a baking dish, place the cooked onion and top with the egg mixture, followed by trout.
5. Select "Air Fry" of Breville Smart Air Fryer Oven and adjust the temperature to 320 degrees F.
6. Set the timer for 20 minutes and press "Start/Stop" to start preheating.
7. When the unit beeps to point out that it's preheated, arrange the baking dish over the wire rack.
8. When the Cooking time is completed, remove the baking dish from oven and place onto a wire rack to chill for about 5 minutes before serving.
9. Cut into equal-sized wedges and serve with the garnishing of dill.

Tomato Quiche

Servings: 2

Preparation time: 15 minutes

Cooking time: 30 minutes

Ingredients:

- 4 eggs
- ¼ cup of onion, chopped
- ½ cup of tomatoes, chopped
- ½ cup of unsweetened almond milk
- 1 cup of low-fat Gouda cheese, shredded Salt, as required

Instructions:

1. In a small baking dish, add all the Ingredients and blend well.
2. Select "Air Fry" of Breville Smart Air Fryer Oven and adjust the temperature to 340 degrees F.
3. Set the timer for 30 minutes and press "Start/Stop" to start preheating.
4. When the unit beeps to point out that it's preheated, arrange the baking dish over the wire rack.

5. When the Cooking time is completed, remove the baking dish from oven and place onto a wire rack to chill for about 5 minutes before serving.

6. Cut into equal-sized wedges and serve.

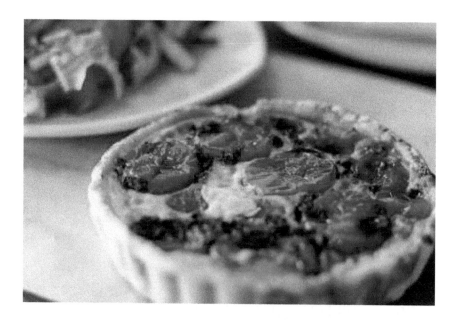

Spinach Quiche

Servings: 4

Preparation time: 10 minutes

Cooking time: 4 hours

Ingredients:

- 10 ounces of frozen chopped spinach, thawed and squeezed
- 4 ounces of feta cheese, shredded
- 2 cups of unsweetened almond milk
- 4 eggs
- ¼ teaspoon of red pepper flakes, crushed
- Salt and ground black pepper, as required

Instructions:

1. In a baking dish, add all the Ingredients and blend until well combined.
2. Arrange the baking dish over the wire rack.
3. Select "Slow Cooker" of Breville Smart Air Fryer Oven and assail "Low".

4. Set the timer for 4 hours and press "Start/Stop" to start cooking.
5. When the Cooking time is completed, remove the baking dish from the oven and transfer the quiche onto a platter.
6. Cut into equal-sized wedges and serve hot.

Chicken & Spinach Quiche

Servings: 4

Preparation time: 15 minutes

Cooking time: 12 minutes

Ingredients:

- 2 ounces of cooked chicken, chopped
- ½ cup of fresh spinach, chopped
- ¼ cup of part-skim mozzarella cheese, shredded
- ½ cup of low-fat Parmesan cheese, shredded
- 2 tablespoons of unsweetened almond milk
- Salt and ground black pepper, as required

Instructions:

1. In a bowl, add all Ingredients and blend well.
2. Transfer the mixture into a baking dish.
3. Select "Air Fry" of Breville Smart Air Fryer Oven and adjust the temperature to 320 degrees F.
4. Set the timer for 12 minutes and press "Start/Stop" to start preheating.

5. When the unit beeps to point out that it's preheated, arrange the baking dish over the wire rack.

6. When the Cooking time is completed, remove the baking dish from oven and place onto a wire rack to chill for about 5 minutes before serving.

7. Cut into equal-sized wedges and serve hot.

Ground Chicken & Mushroom Frittata

Servings: 4

Preparation time: 15 minutes

Cooking time: 40 minutes

Ingredients:

- 2 tablespoons of olive oil, divided
- 8 ounces of ground chicken
- 8 ounces of fresh mushrooms, chopped
- 8 eggs
- 3 tablespoons of coconut cream
- 3 tablespoons of fresh parsley, chopped
- ¼ teaspoon of garlic powder
- Salt and ground black pepper, as required
- ½ cup of low-fat cheddar cheese, shredded

Instructions:

1. In a skillet, heat 1 tablespoon of oil over medium-high heat and cook the ground chicken for about 5 minutes, stirring frequently and ending the meat.

2. With a slotted spoon, place the cooked chicken into a bowl.

3. In the same skillet, heat the remaining tablespoon of oil over medium heat and cook the mushrooms for about 10 minutes, stirring occasionally.

4. Transfer the mushrooms into the bowl with cooked chicken and put aside to chill.

5. In a large bowl, add the eggs, coconut milk, parsley, thyme, onion powder, garlic powder, salt and black pepper and beat until well combined.

6. Add the cheese and stir to mix.

7. Add the chicken mixture and blend well.

8. Place the mixture into a greased baking pan.

9. Arrange the pan over the wire rack.

10. Select "Bake" of Breville Smart Air Fryer Oven and adjust the temperature to 325 degrees F.

11. Set the timer for 25 minutes and press "Start/Stop" to start preheating.

12. When the unit beeps to point out that it's preheated, insert the wire rack in the oven.

13. When the Cooking time is completed, remove the pan from the oven and put aside to chill for five minutes before serving.

Salmon Quiche

Servings: 2

Preparation time: 15 minutes

Cooking time: 20 minutes

Ingredients:

- 5½ ounces of salmon fillet, chopped
- Salt and ground black pepper, as required
- ½ tablespoon of fresh lemon juice
- 1 egg yolk
- 3½ tablespoons of chilled coconut oil
- 2/3 cups of flour
- 1 tablespoon of cold water
- 2 eggs
- 3 tablespoons of whipping cream
- 1 scallion, chopped

Instructions:

1. In a bowl, add the salmon, salt, black pepper and juice and blend well.
2. In another bowl, add the ingredient, coconut oil, flour and water and blend until a dough forms.
3. Place the dough onto a floured smooth surface and roll into about 7-inch round.
4. Place the dough in a quiche pan and press firmly in the bottom and along the sides.
5. Trim the surplus edges.
6. In a small bowl, add the eggs, cream, salt and black pepper and beat until well combined.
7. Place the cream mixture over the crust evenly and top with the salmon mixture, followed by the scallion.
8. Select "Air Fry" of Breville Smart Air Fryer Oven and adjust the temperature to 355 degrees F.
9. Set the timer for 20 minutes and press "Start/Stop" to start preheating.
10. When the unit beeps to point out that it's preheated, arrange the quiche pan over the wire rack.
11. When the Cooking time is completed, remove the quiche pan from the oven and put aside for about 5 minutes before serving.
12. Cut the quiche into equal-sized wedges and serve.

Beef & Mushroom Casserole

Servings: 6

Preparation time: 15 minutes

Cooking time: 19 minutes

Ingredients:

- 1 tablespoon of olive oil
- ½ pound ground beef
- ¾ cup of yellow onion, chopped
- 5 fresh mushrooms, sliced
- 8 eggs, beaten
- ½ teaspoon of garlic salt
- ¾ cup of low-fat Cheddar cheese, shredded and divided
- ¼ cup of sugar-free Alfredo sauce

Instructions:

1. In a skillet, heat the oil over medium heat and cook the meat and onions for about 4-5 minutes.
2. Add the mushrooms and cook for about 6-7 minutes.
3. Remove from the oven and drain the grease from the skillet.

4. In a bowl, add the meat mixture, beaten eggs, garlic salt, ½ cup of cheese and Alfredo sauce and stir to mix.
5. Place the meat mixture into a baking dish.
6. Select "Air Fry" of Breville Smart Air Fryer Oven and adjust the temperature to 390 degrees F.
7. Set the timer for 12 minutes and press "Start/Stop" to start preheating.
8. When the unit beeps to point out that it's preheated, arrange the baking dish over the wire rack.
9. After 6 minutes of cooking, stir the sausage mixture well.
10. When the Cooking time is completed, remove the baking dish from oven and place onto a wire rack to chill for about 5 minutes before serving.
11. Cut into equal-sized wedges and serve with the topping of remaining cheese.

Chicken & Cauliflower Casserole

Servings: 5

Preparation time: 15 minutes

Cooking time: 35 minutes

Ingredients:

- 1½ tablespoons of olive oil
- ½ of large onion, chopped
- 24 ounces of cauliflower rice
- 3 eggs
- 2 tablespoons of unsweetened almond milk
- Salt and ground black pepper, as required
- ½ pound cooked chicken, chopped
- ¼ cup of low-fat Cheddar cheese, shredded

Instructions:

1. In a skillet, heat the oil over medium heat and sauté the onion for about 4-5 minutes.
2. Remove from the heat and transfer the onion into a bowl.
3. Add the cauliflower rice and blend well.
4. Place the mixture into a baking dish.

5. Select "Bake" of Breville Smart Air Fryer Oven and adjust the temperature to 350 degrees F.

6. Set the timer for 32 minutes and press "Start/Stop" to start preheating.

7. When the unit beeps to point out that it's preheated, arrange the baking dish over the wire rack.

8. Stir the mixture once after 8 minutes.

9. Meanwhile, in a bowl, add the eggs, milk, salt and black pepper and beat well.

10. After 15 minutes of cooking, place the egg mixture over cauliflower rice mixture evenly and top with the chicken pieces.

11. After 30 minutes of cooking, sprinkle the casserole with the cheese.

12. When the Cooking time is completed, remove the baking dish from oven and place onto a wire rack to chill for about 5 minutes before serving.

13. Cut into equal-sized wedges and serve.

Eggs with Turkey & Spinach

Servings: 4

Preparation time: 15 minutes

Cooking time: 23 minutes

Ingredients:

- 1 tablespoon of coconut oil
- 1-pound fresh baby spinach
- 4 eggs
- 7 ounces of cooked turkey, chopped
- 4 teaspoons of unsweetened almond milk
- Salt and ground black pepper, as required

Instructions:

1. In a skillet, melt the coconut oil over medium heat and cook the spinach for about 2-3 minutes or until just wilted.
2. Remove from the heat and transfer the spinach into a bowl.
3. Put aside to chill slightly.

4. Divide the spinach into 4 greased ramekins, followed by the turkey.
5. Crack 1 egg into each ramekin and drizzle with almond milk.
6. Sprinkle with salt and black pepper.
7. Select "Air Fry" of Breville Smart Air Fryer Oven and adjust the temperature to 355 degrees F.
8. Set the timer for 20 minutes and press "Start/Stop" to start preheating.
9. When the unit beeps to point out that it's preheated, arrange the ramekins over the wire rack.
10. When the Cooking time is completed, remove the ramekins from oven and place onto a wire rack to chill for about 5 minutes before serving.

Eggs with Turkey

Servings: 2

Preparation time: 10 minutes

Cooking time: 13 minutes

Ingredients:

- 2 teaspoons of coconut oil, softened
- 2 ounces of cooked turkey breast, sliced thinly
- 4 large eggs, divided
- 1 tablespoon of coconut milk
- Salt and ground black pepper, as required
- 1/8 teaspoon of smoked paprika
- 3 tablespoons of low-fat Parmesan cheese, grated finely
- 2 teaspoons of fresh chives, minced

Instructions:

1. In the bottom of a baking dish, spread the coconut oil.
2. Arrange the turkey slices over the coconut oil.
3. In a bowl, add 1egg, coconut milk, salt and black pepper and beat until smooth.
4. Place the egg mixture over the turkey slices evenly.

5. Carefully crack the remaining eggs on top and sprinkle with paprika, salt, black pepper, cheese and chives evenly.

6. Select "Air Fry" of Breville Smart Air Fryer Oven and adjust the temperature to 320 degrees F.

7. Set the timer for 13 minutes and press "Start/Stop" to start preheating.

8. When the unit beeps to point out that it's preheated, arrange the baking dish over the wire rack.

9. When the Cooking time is completed, remove the baking dish from the oven and put aside for about 5 minutes before serving.

10. Cut into equal-sized wedges and serve.

Cranberry Muffins

Servings: 8

Preparation time: 25 minutes

Cooking time: 15 minutes

Ingredients:

- ¼ cup of unsweetened almond milk
- 2 large eggs
- ½ teaspoon of vanilla extract
- 1½ cups of almond flour
- ¼ cup of Erythritol
- 1 teaspoon of baking powder
- ¼ teaspoon of ground cinnamon
- 1/8 teaspoon of salt
- ½ cup of fresh cranberries
- ¼ cup of walnuts, chopped

Instructions:

1. In a blender, add the almond milk, eggs, vanilla, and pulse for about 20-30 seconds.

2. Add the almond flour, Erythritol, baking powder, cinnamon, salt, and pulse for about 30-45 seconds until well blended.

3. Transfer the mixture into a bowl.

4. Gently fold in half the cranberries and walnuts.

5. Place the mixture into 8 silicone muffin cups of and top each with remaining cranberries.

6. Select "Air Fry" of Breville Smart Air Fryer Oven and adjust the temperature to 325 degrees F.

7. Set the timer for 15 minutes and press "Start/Stop" to start preheating.

8. When the unit beeps to point out that it's preheated, arrange the muffin cups of over the wire rack.

9. When the Cooking time is completed, remove the muffin cups of from oven and place onto a wire rack to chill for about 10 minutes.

10. Carefully invert the muffins onto the wire rack to completely cool before serving.

Savory Carrot Muffins

Servings: 6

Preparation time: 15 minutes

Cooking time: 7 minutes

Ingredients:

For Muffins:

- ¼ cup of whole-wheat flour
- ¼ cup of all-purpose flour
- ½ teaspoon of baking powder
- 1/8 teaspoon of baking soda
- ½ teaspoon of dried parsley, crushed
- ½ teaspoon of salt
- ½ cup of low-fat plain yoghurt
- 1 teaspoon of vinegar
- 1 tablespoon of olive oil
- 3 tablespoons of cottage cheese, grated
- 1 carrot, peeled and grated
- 2-4 tablespoons of water (if needed)

For Topping:

- 7 ounces of low-fat Parmesan cheese, grated
- ¼ cup of walnuts, chopped

Instructions:

1. For muffins: in a large bowl, mix together the flours, baking powder, baking soda, parsley, and salt.
2. In another large bowl, add the yoghurt and vinegar and blend well.
3. Add the remaining Ingredients apart from water and beat them well. (Add some water if needed).
4. Make a well in the centre of the yoghurt mixture.
5. Slowly add the flour mixture in the well and blend until well combined.
6. Place the mixture into lightly greased 6 medium-sized muffin molds evenly and top with the Parmesan cheese and walnuts.
7. Select "Air Fry" of Breville Smart Air Fryer Oven and adjust the temperature to 355 degrees F.
8. Set the timer for 7 minutes and press "Start/Stop" to start preheating.
9. When the unit beeps to point out that it's preheated, arrange the muffin molds over the wire rack.
10. When the Cooking time is completed, remove the muffin molds from the oven and place onto a wire rack to chill for about 5 minutes.

11. Carefully invert the muffins onto the platter and serve warm.

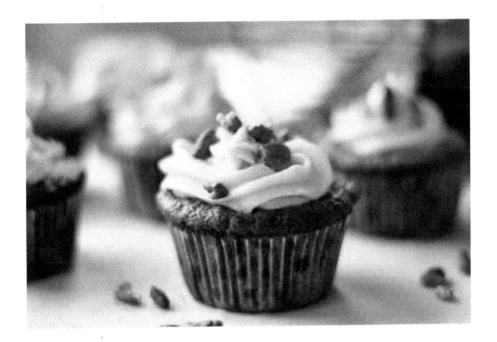

Chicken & Spinach Muffins

Servings: 6

Preparation time: 10 minutes

Cooking time: 17 minutes

Ingredients:

- 6 eggs
- ½ cup of unsweetened almond milk
- Salt and ground black pepper, as required
- 2 ounces of cooked chicken, chopped
- ¾ cup of fresh spinach, chopped

Instructions:

1. In a bowl, add the eggs, milk, salt and black pepper and beat until well combined.
2. Add the chicken and spinach and stir to mix.
3. Divide the spinach mixture into 6 greased cups of an egg bite mold evenly.
4. Select "Air Fry" of Breville Smart Air Fryer Oven and adjust the temperature to 325 degrees F.

5. Set the timer for 17 minutes and press "Start/Stop" to start preheating.

6. When the unit beeps to point out that it's preheated, arrange the egg bite mold over the wire rack.

7. When the Cooking time is completed, remove the egg bite mold from oven and place onto a wire rack to chill for about 5 minutes.

8. Serve warm.

Zucchini Fritters

Servings: 4

Preparation time: 15 minutes

Cooking time: 7 minutes

Ingredients:

- 10½ ounces of zucchini, grated and squeezed
- 7 ounces of low-fat Halloumi cheese
- ¼ cup of almond flour
- 2 eggs
- 1 teaspoon of fresh dill, minced
- Salt and ground black pepper, as required

Instructions:

1. In a large bowl and blend together all the Ingredients.
2. Make small-sized fritters from the mixture.
3. Arrange the fritters into the greased enamel roasting pan.
4. Select "Air Fry" of Breville Smart Air Fryer Oven and adjust the temperature to 355 degrees F.
5. Set the timer for 7 minutes and press "Start/Stop" to start preheating.

6. When the unit beeps to point out that it's preheated, insert the roasting pan in the oven.

7. When the Cooking time is completed, remove the roasting pan from the oven.

8. Serve warm.

Onion Soup

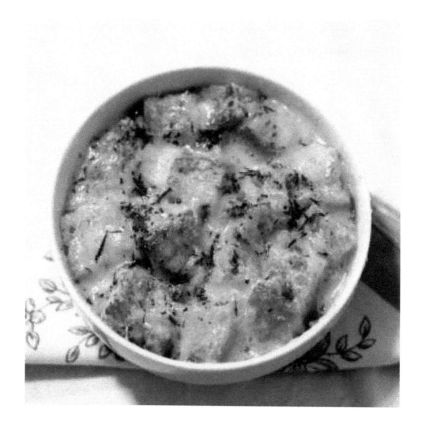

Servings: 6

Preparation time: 15 minutes

Cooking time: 5 hours 10 minutes

Ingredients:

- 2 tablespoons of olive oil
- 2 medium sweet onions, sliced

- 2 garlic cloves, minced
- ¼ cup of low-sodium soy sauce
- 1 teaspoon of unsweetened applesauce
- 1 teaspoon of dried oregano, crushed
- 1 teaspoon of dried basil, crushed
- Ground black pepper, as required
- 5 cups of low-sodium vegetable broth
- ¼ cup of low-fat Parmesan cheese, grated

Instructions:

1. In an oven-safe pan that will put in the Breville Smart Air Fryer Oven, heat the oil over medium heat and cook the onion for about 8-9 minutes.
2. Add the garlic and cook for about 1 minute.
3. Remove from the heat and stir in the remaining Ingredients apart from cheese.
4. Cover the pan with a lid.
5. Arrange the pan over the wire rack.
6. Select "Slow Cooker" of Breville Smart Air Fryer Oven and assail "Low".
7. Set the timer for five hours and press "Start/Stop" to start cooking.
8. When the Cooking time is completed, remove the pan from the oven.

9. Remove the lid and stir in the cheese until melted completely.
10. Serve hot.

Mixed Veggies Soup

Servings: 6

Preparation time: 15 minutes

Cooking time: 8 hours 5 minutes

Ingredients:

- 1 tablespoon of olive oil
- 1 yellow onion, chopped
- 1 celery stalk, chopped
- 1 large carrot, peeled and chopped
- 2 garlic cloves, minced
- 1 teaspoon of dried oregano, crushed
- 1 large zucchini, chopped
- 2 tomatoes, chopped
- 1 cup of fresh spinach, chopped
- 4 cups of homemade low-sodium vegetable broth
- Salt and ground black pepper, as required

Instructions:

1. In an oven-safe pan that will put in the Breville Smart Air Fryer Oven, heat the oil over medium heat and sauté the onion, celery and carrot for about 3-4 minutes.
2. Add the garlic, thyme, and sauté for about 1 minute.
3. Remove from the heat and stir in the remaining Ingredients.
4. Cover the pan with a lid.
5. Arrange the pan over the wire rack.
6. Select "Slow Cooker" of Breville Smart Air Fryer Oven and assail "Low".
7. Set the timer for 8 hours and press "Start/Stop" to start cooking.
8. When the Cooking time is completed, remove the pan from the oven.
9. Remove the lid and stir the mixture well.
10. Serve hot.

Lean and green Pizza Hack

Preparation time: 5-10 minutes

Cooking time: 15-20 minutes

Servings: 1

Ingredients:

- 1/4 fueling of garlic mashed potato
- 1/2 egg whites
- 1/4 tablespoon of baking powder
- 3/4 oz. of reduced-fat shredded mozzarella
- 1/8 cup of sliced white mushrooms
- 1/16 cup of pizza sauce
- 3/4 oz. of ground beef
- 1/4 sliced black olives

You also need a sauté pan, baking sheets, and parchment paper

Directions:

1. Start by preheating the oven to 400°F.
2. Mix your baking powder and garlic potato packet.

3. Add egg whites to your mixture and stir well until it blends.
4. Line the baking sheet with parchment paper and pour the mixed batter onto it.
5. Put another parchment paper on top of the batter and open up the batter to a 1/8-inch circle.
6. Then place another baking sheet on top; this way, the batter is between two baking sheets.
7. Place in an oven and bake for about 8 minutes until the pizza crust is golden brown.
8. For the toppings, place your hamburger in a sauté pan and fry till it's brown, and then wash your mushrooms thoroughly.
9. After the crust is baked, remove the top layer of parchment paper carefully to prevent the froth from sticking to the pizza crust.
10. Put your toppings on top of the crust and bake for an additional 8 minutes.
11. Once ready, slide the pizza off the parchment paper and onto a plate.

Nutrition:

- Calories: 478
- Protein: 30 g
- Carbohydrates: 22 g

- Fats: 29 g

Amaranth Porridge

Preparation time: 5 minutes

Cooking time: 30 minutes

Servings: 2

Ingredients:

- 2 cups of coconut milk
- 2 cups of alkaline water
- 1 cup of amaranth
- 2 tbsps. Of coconut oil
- 1 tbsp. of ground cinnamon

Directions:

1. In a saucepan, mix in the milk with water, then boil the mixture.
2. Stir in the amaranth, then reduce the heat to medium.
3. Cook on the medium heat, then simmer for a minimum of 30 minutes while stirring occasionally.

4. Turn off the heat.

5. Add in cinnamon and coconut oil then stir.

6. Serve.

Nutrition:

- Calories: 434
- Fat: 35 g
- Carbs: 27 g
- Protein: 6.7 g

Lavender Blueberry Chia Seed Pudding

Preparation time: 1 hour 10 minutes

Cooking time: 0 minutes

Servings: 4

Ingredients:

- 100 g of blueberries
- 70 g of organic quark
- 50 g of soy yogurt
- 30 g of hazelnuts
- 200 ml of almond milk
- 2 tbsp. of chia seeds
- 2 teaspoons of agave syrup
- 2 teaspoons of lavender

Directions:

1. Bring the almond milk to a boil alongside the lavender.
2. Let the mixture simmer for 10 minutes at a reduced temperature.

3. Let them calm down afterwards.
4. If the milk is cold, add the blueberries and puree everything.
5. Mix the entire thing with the chia seeds and agave syrup.
6. Let everything soak in the refrigerator for an hour.
7. Mix the yogurt and curd cheese together.
8. Add both to the group.
9. Divide the pudding into glasses.
10. Finely chop the hazelnuts and sprinkle them on top.

Nutrition:

- Kcal: 252
- Carbohydrates: 12 g
- Protein: 1 g
- Fat: 11 g

Coconut Chia Pudding with Berries

Preparation time: 20 minutes

Cooking time: 45 minutes

Servings: 2

Ingredients:

- 150 g of raspberries and blueberries
- 60 g of chia seeds
- 500 ml of coconut milk
- 1 teaspoon of agave syrup
- ½ teaspoon of ground bourbon vanilla

Directions:

1. Put the chia seeds, agave syrup, and vanilla in a bowl.
2. Pour in the coconut milk.
3. Mix thoroughly and let it soak for 30 minutes.
4. Meanwhile, wash the berries and allow them to drain well.
5. Divide the coconut chia pudding between two glasses.

6. Put the berries on top.

Nutrition:

- Kcal: 662
- Carbohydrates: 18 g
- Protein: 8 g
- Fat: 55 g

Omelette with Tomatoes and Spring Onions

Preparation time: 5 minutes

Cooking time: 20 minutes

Ingredients:

- 6 eggs
- 2 tomatoes
- 2 spring onions
- 1 shallot
- 2 tbsps. of butter
- 1 tbsp. of olive oil
- 1 pinch of nutmeg salt
- Pepper

Directions:

1. Whisk the eggs in a bowl.
2. Mix them together and season them with salt and pepper.
3. Peel the shallot and chop it up.
4. Clean the onions and cut them into rings.

5. Wash the tomatoes and cut them into pieces.

6. Heat butter and oil in a pan.

7. Braise half the shallots in it.

8. Add half the egg mixture.

9. Let everything set over medium heat.

10. Scatter a couple of tomatoes and onion rings on top.

11. Repeat with the last half of the egg mixture.

12. At the end, spread the grated nutmeg over the entire thing.

Nutrition:

- Kcal: 263
- Carbohydrates: 8 g
- Protein: 20.3 g
- Fat: 24 g

Bacon Cheeseburger

Preparation time: 5 minutes

Cooking time: 15 minutes

Servings: 4

Ingredients:

- 1 lb. of lean ground beef
- ¼ cup of chopped yellow onion
- 1 clove of garlic, minced
- 1 tbsp. of yellow mustard
- 1 tbsp. of Worcestershire sauce
- ½ tsp. of salt
- Cooking spray
- 4 ultra-thin slices of cheddar cheese, cut into 6 equal-sized rectangular pieces
- 3 pieces of turkey bacon, each cut into 8 evenly-sized rectangular pieces
- 24 dill pickle chips
- 4-6 green leaf lettuce leaves, torn into 24 small square-shaped pieces
- 12 cherry tomatoes; sliced in half

Directions:

1. Pre-heat oven to 400°F.
2. Combine the garlic, salt, onion, Worcester sauce, and beef in a medium-sized bowl, and blend well.
3. Form mixture into 24 small meatballs. Place meatballs onto a foil-lined baking sheet and cook for 12-15 minutes. Leave oven on.
4. Top every meatball with a bit of cheese, then return to the oven till cheese melts, about 2 to 3 minutes. Let meatballs cool.
5. To assemble bites: on a toothpick, layer a cheese-covered meatball, piece of bacon, piece of lettuce, pickle chip, and a tomato half.

Nutrition:

- Calories: 234
- Protein: 20 g
- Fat: 3 g
- Carbs: 12 g

Chia Seed Gel with Pomegranate and Nuts

Preparation time: 5 minutes

Cooking time: 10 minutes

Servings: 3

Ingredients:

- 20 g of hazelnuts
- 20 g of walnuts
- 120 ml of almond milk
- 4 tbsps. of chia seeds
- 4 tbsps. of pomegranate seeds
- 1 teaspoon of agave syrup
- Some lime juices

Directions:

1. Finely chop the nuts.
2. Mix the almond milk with the chia seeds. Let everything soak for 10 to 20 minutes.
3. Occasionally stir the mixture with the chia seeds.

4. Stir in the agave syrup.
5. Pour 2 tablespoons of every mixture into a dessert glass.
6. Layer the chopped nuts on top.
7. Cover the nuts with 1 tablespoon each of the chia mass.
8. Sprinkle the pomegranate seeds on top and serve everything.

Nutrition:

- Kcal: 248
- Carbohydrates: 7 g
- Protein: 1 g
- Fat: 19 g

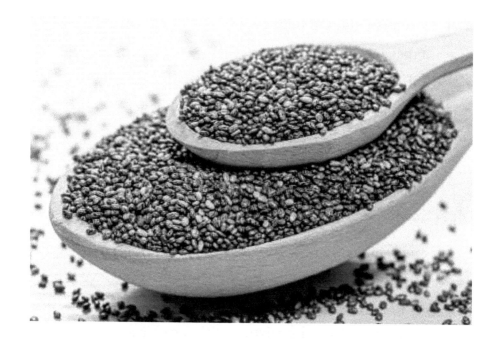

Pancakes with Berries

Preparation time: 5 minutes

Cooking time: 20 minutes

Servings: 2

Ingredients:

Pancake:

- 1 egg
- 50 g of spelled flour
- 50 g of almond flour
- 15 g of coconut flour
- 150 ml of water salt

Filling:

- 40 g of mixed berries
- 10 g of chocolate
- 5 g of powdered sugar
- 4 tbsps. of yogurt

Directions:

1. Put the flour, egg, and a few salt in a blender jar.

2. Add 150 ml of water.

3. Mix everything with a whisk.

4. Mix everything into a batter.

5. Heat a coated pan.

6. Put in half the batter.

7. Once the pancake is firm, turn it over.

8. Take out the pancake, then add the last half of the batter to the pan and repeat.

9. Melt chocolate over a water bath.

10. Let the pancakes cool.

11. Brush the pancakes with the yogurt.

12. Wash the berry and let it drain.

13. Put berries on the yogurt.

14. Roll up the pancakes.

15. Sprinkle them with the granulated sugar.

16. Decorate the entire thing with the melted chocolate.

Nutrition:

- Kcal: 298
- Carbohydrates: 26 g
- Protein: 21 g
- Fat: 9 g

Porridge with Walnuts

Preparation time: 5 minutes

Cooking time: 10 minutes

Servings: 1

Ingredients:

- 50 g of raspberries
- 50 g of blueberries
- 25 g of ground walnuts
- 20 g of crushed flaxseed
- 10 g of oatmeal
- 200 ml of nut drink
- Agave syrup
- ½ teaspoon of cinnamon salt

Directions:

1. Heat the nut drink a little in a saucepan.
2. Add the walnuts, flaxseed, and oatmeal, stirring constantly.
3. Stir in the cinnamon and salt.
4. Simmer for 8 minutes.

5. Keep stirring everything.

6. Sweet the entire mixture.

7. Put the porridge in a bowl.

8. Wash the berries and allow them to drain.

9. Add them to the porridge and serve everything.

Nutrition:

- Kcal: 378
- Carbohydrates: 11 g
- Protein: 18 g
- Fat: 27 g

Omelette à la Margherita

Preparation time: 10 minutes

Cooking time: 20 minutes

Servings: 2

Ingredients:

- 3 eggs
- 50 g of parmesan cheese
- 2 tbsps. of heavy cream
- 1 tbsp. of olive oil
- 1 teaspoon of oregano nutmeg
- Salt
- Pepper
- For covering:
- 3-4 stalks of basil
- 1 tomato
- 100 g of grated mozzarella

Directions:

1. Mix the cream and eggs in a medium bowl.

2. Add the grated parmesan, nutmeg, oregano, pepper and salt, and stir everything.
3. Heat the oil in a pan.
4. Add 1/2 of the egg and cream to the pan.
5. Let the omelet set over medium heat, turn it, then remove it.
6. Repeat with the last half of the egg mixture.
7. Cut the tomatoes into slices and place them on top of the omelets.
8. Scatter the mozzarella over the tomatoes.
9. Place the omelets on a baking sheet.
10. Cook at 180 degrees for 5 to 10 minutes.
11. Then take the omelets out and decorate them with the basil leaves.

Nutrition:

- Kcal: 402
- Carbohydrates: 7 g
- Protein: 21 g
- Fat: 34 g

Sweet Cashew Cheese Spread

Preparation time: 5 minutes

Cooking time: 5 minutes

Servings: 10

Ingredients:

- Stevia (5 drops)
- Cashews (2 cups, raw)
- Water (1/2 cup)

Directions:

1. Soak the cashews in water overnight.
2. Next, drain the surplus water then transfer cashews to a food processor.
3. Add in the stevia and the water.
4. Process until smooth.
5. Serve chilled. Enjoy.

Nutrition:

- Fat: 7 g

- Cholesterol: 0 mg
- Sodium: 12.6 mg
- Carbohydrates: 5.7 g

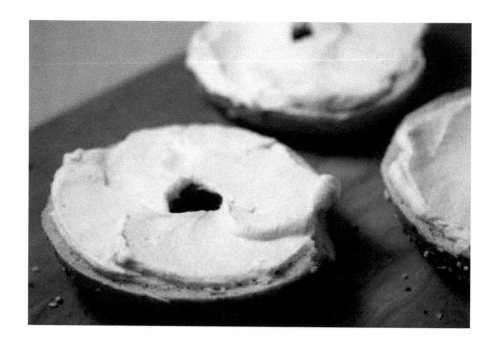

Personal Biscuit Pizza

Preparation time: 5 minutes

Cooking time: 15 minutes

Servings: 1

Ingredients:

- 1 sachet of LEAN AND GREEN Select
- Buttermilk Cheddar Herb Biscuit
- 2 tbsp. of cold water
- Cooking spray
- 2 tbsp. of no-sugar-added tomato sauce
- ¼ cup of reduced-fat shredded cheese

Directions:

1. Preheat oven to 350°F.
2. Mix biscuit and water, and spread mixture into a little, circular crust shape onto a greased, foil-lined baking sheet. Bake for 10 minutes.
3. Top with spaghetti sauce and cheese, and cook till cheese is melted, about 5 minutes.

Nutrition:

- Calories: 301
- Protein: 13 g
- Fat: 8
- Carbs: 7

Fried Egg with Bacon

Preparation time: 5 minutes

Cooking time: 10 minutes

Servings: 1

Ingredients:

- 2 eggs
- 30 grams of bacon
- 2 tbsps. of olive oil salt
- Pepper

Directions:

1. Heat oil in the pan and fry the bacon.
2. Reduce the heat and beat the eggs in the pan.
3. Cook the eggs and season with salt and pepper.
4. Serve the fried eggs hot with the bacon.

Nutrition:

- Kcal: 405
- Carbohydrates: 1 g
- Protein: 19 g
- Fat: 38 g

Eel on Scrambled Eggs and Bread

Preparation time: 5 minutes

Cooking time: 10 minutes

Servings: 2

Ingredients:

- 4 eggs
- 1 shallot
- 4 slices of low carb bread
- 2 sticks of dill
- 200 g of smoked eel
- 1 tbsp. of oil
- Salt
- White pepper

Directions:

1. Mix the eggs in a bowl and season with salt and pepper.
2. Peel the shallot and cut it into fine cubes.
3. Chop the dill.

4. Remove the skin from the eel and cut it into pieces.

5. Heat the oil in a pan and steam the shallot in it.

6. Add in the eggs and allow them to set.

7. Use the spatula to stir the eggs several times.

8. Reduce the heat and add the dill.

9. Stir everything.

10. Spread the scrambled eggs over four slices of bread.

11. Put the eel pieces on top.

12. Add some fresh dill and serve everything.

Nutrition:

- Kcal: 830
- Carbohydrates: 8 g
- Protein: 45 g
- Fat: 64 g

Whole Grain Bread and Avocado

Preparation time: 5 minutes

Cooking time: 0 minutes

Serving: 1

Ingredients:

- 2 slices of whole meal bread
- 60 g of cottage cheese
- 1 stick of thyme
- ½ avocado
- ½ lime Chili flakes
- Salt
- Pepper

Directions:

1. Cut the avocado in half.
2. Remove the pulp and cut it into slices.
3. Pour the juice over it.
4. Wash the thyme and shake it dry.
5. Remove the leaves from the stem.
6. Brush the entire wheat bread with the pot cheese.

7. Place the avocado slices on top.

8. Top with the chili flakes and thyme.

9. Add salt and pepper and serve.

Nutrition:

- Kcal: 490
- Carbohydrates: 31 g
- Protein: 19 g
- Fat: 21 g

Cheeseburger Pie

Preparation time: 25 minutes

Cooking time: 90 minutes

Servings: 4

Ingredients:

- 1 large spaghetti squash
- 1 lb. of lean ground beef
- ¼ cup of diced onion
- 2 eggs
- 1/3 cup of low-fat, plain Greek yogurt
- 2 Tbsp. of Tomato sauce
- ½ tsp. of Worcestershire sauce
- 2/3 cup of reduced-fat, shredded cheddar cheese
- 2 oz. of dill pickle slices
- Cooking spray

Directions:

1. Preheat oven to 400°F.
2. Slice spaghetti squash in half lengthwise; throw out pulp and seeds. Spray with cooking spray.

3. Place the cut pumpkin halves on a foil-lined baking sheet and bake for 30 minutes. Once cooked, let it cool before scraping the pulp from the squash with a fork to get rid of the spaghetti-like strings. Set aside.

4. Push squash strands in the bottom and up sides of the greased pie pan, creating a good layer.

5. Meanwhile, set up pie filling. In a lightly greased, medium-sized skillet, cook beef and onion over medium heat for 8 to 10 minutes, sometimes stirring, until meat is brown. Drain and take away from heat. Whisk together the eggs, tomato paste, Greek yogurt, Worcester sauce, and add the ground beef mixture. Pour the pie filling over the pumpkin rind.

1. Sprinkle the meat filling with cheese, then fill with pickled cucumber slices.

2. Bake for 40 minutes.

Nutrition:

- Calories: 270
- Protein: 23 g
- Carbohydrate: 10 g
- Fat: 23 g

Asparagus & Crabmeat Frittata

Preparation time: 5 minutes

Cooking time: 15 minutes

Servings: 4

Ingredients:

- 2½ tbsp. of extra virgin olive oil
- 2 lbs. of asparagus
- 1 tsp. of salt
- 1 ½ tsp. of black pepper
- 2 tsps. of sweet paprika
- 1 lb. of lump crabmeat
- 1 tbsp. of finely cut chives
- ¼ cup of basil chopped
- 4 cups of liquid egg substitute

Directions:

1. Remove the tough ends of the asparagus and cut it into bite-sized pieces.
2. Preheat an oven to 375°F.

3. In a 12-Inch to a 14-inch oven-proof, non-stick skillet, warm the vegetable oil and boil the asparagus until soft. Season with pepper, paprika, and salt.

4. In a bowl, add the chives, crab and basil meat.

5. Pour in the liquid egg substitute and blend until it has combined.

6. Pour the crab and egg mixture into the skillet with the cooked asparagus and stir to mix. Bake over low to medium heat until the eggs start bubbling.

7. Place the skillet in the oven and bake for about 15-20 minutes until the eggs are golden brown. Serve the dish warm.

Nutrition:

- Calories: 340
- Protein: 50 g
- Carbohydrate: 14 g
- Fat: 10g

Grilled Chicken Power Bowl with Green Goddess Dressing

Preparation time: 5 minutes

Cooking time: 15 minutes

Servings: 4

Ingredients:

- 1 ½ boneless, skinless chicken breasts
- ¼ tsp. each of salt & pepper
- 1 cup of diced or cubed kabocha squash
- 1 cup of diced zucchini
- 1 cup of diced yellow summer squash
- 1 cup of diced broccoli
- 8 cherry tomatoes, halved
- 4 radishes, sliced thin
- 1 cup of shredded red cabbage
- ¼ cup of hemp or pumpkin seeds Green Goddess Dressing:
- ½ cup of low-fat plain Greek yogurt
- 1 cup of fresh basil
- 1 clove of garlic
- 4 tbsps. of lemon juice

- ¼ tsp. of each salt & pepper

Directions:

1. Pre-heat oven to 350°F.
2. Season chicken with salt and pepper.
3. Roast chicken for 12 minutes until it reaches a temperature of 165°F. When done, remove from oven and put aside to rest, about 5 minutes. Cut in bite-sized pieces and keep warm.
4. While the chicken rests, steam diced kabocha squash, yellow summer squash, zucchini, and broccoli in a covered microwave-proof bowl for about 5 minutes, till soft.
5. For the dressing, arrange the Ingredients in a blender and puree till smooth.
6. To serve, place an equal amount of Veggie Mix into four individual bowls. Add an equal amount of cherry tomatoes, radishes, and chopped cabbage to every bowl alongside 1/4 of the chicken and a tablespoon of seeds.
7. Dress up. Enjoy!

Nutrition:

- Calories: 300
- Protein: 43 g
- Carbohydrate: 12 g

- Fat: 10 g

Yogurt with Granola and Persimmon

Preparation time: 5 minutes

Cooking time: 5 minutes

Servings: 1

Ingredients:

- 150 g of Greek style yogurt
- 20 g of oatmeal
- 60 g of fresh persimmons
- 30 ml of tap water

Directions:

1. Put the oatmeal in the pan with no fat.
2. Toast them, stirring constantly, until golden brown.
3. Then put them on a plate and allow them to cool down briefly.
4. Peel the persimmon and put it in a bowl with the water. Mix everything into a fine puree.

5. Put the yogurt, toasted oatmeal, and the puree in layers in a glass and serve.

Nutrition:

- Kcal: 286
- Carbohydrates: 29 g
- Protein: 1 g
- Fat: 11 g

Smoothie Bowl with Spinach, Mango, and Muesli

Preparation time: 10 minutes

Cooking time: 0 minutes

Servings: 1

Ingredients:

- 150 g of yogurt
- 30 g of apple
- 30 g of mango
- 30 g of low carb muesli
- 10 g of spinach
- 10 g of chia seeds

Directions:

1. Soak the spinach leaves and allow them to drain.
2. Peel the mango and cut it into strips.
3. Remove apple core and cut it into pieces.
4. Put everything except the mango alongside the yogurt in a blender and make a fine puree out of them.

5. Put the spinach smoothie in a bowl.

6. Add the muesli, chia seeds, and mango.

7. Serve the whole thing.

Nutrition:

- Kcal: 362
- Carbohydrates: 21 g
- Protein: 12 g
- Fat: 21 g

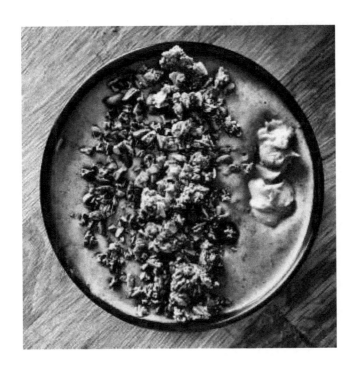

Smoothie Bowl with Berries, Poppy Seeds, Nuts and Seeds

Preparation time: 15 minutes

Cooking time: 0 minutes

Servings: 2

Ingredients:

- 5 chopped almonds
- 2 chopped walnuts
- 1 apple
- ¼ banana
- 300 g of yogurt
- 60 g of raspberries
- 20 g of blueberries
- 20 g of rolled oats; roasted in a pan
- 10 g of poppy seeds
- 1 teaspoon of pumpkin seeds
- Agave syrup

Directions:

1. Clean the fruit and let it drain.
2. Take some berries and set them aside.
3. Place the remaining berries in a tall mixing vessel.
4. Cut the banana into slices, and put a couple of the slices aside.
5. Add the rest of the banana to the berries.
6. Remove the core of the apple and cut it into quarters.
7. Cut the quarters into thin wedges and set a couple of them aside.
8. Add the remaining wedges to the berries.
9. Add the yogurt to the fruits and blend everything into a puree.
10. Sweeten the smoothie with the agave syrup.
11. Divide it into two bowls.
12. Serve it with the remaining fruit, poppy seeds, oatmeal, nuts and seeds.

Nutrition:

- Kcal: 284
- Carbohydrates: 21 g
- Protein: 11 g
- Fat: 19 g

Mini Zucchini Bites

Preparation time: 10 minutes

Cooking time: 10 minutes

Servings: 6

Ingredients:

- 1 zucchini, cut into thick circles
- 3 cherry tomatoes; halved
- 1/2 cup of parmesan cheese; grated
- Salt and pepper to taste
- 1 tsp. of chives; chopped

Directions:

1. Preheat the oven to 3900 F.
2. Add paper on a baking sheet.
3. Arrange the zucchini pieces.
4. Add the cherry halves on each zucchini slice.
5. Add parmesan cheese, chives, and sprinkle with salt and pepper.
6. Bake for 10 minutes. Serve.

Nutrition:

- Fat: 1.0 g
- Cholesterol: 5.0 mg
- Sodium: 400.3 mg
- Potassium: 50.5 mg
- Carbohydrates: 7.3 g

Beef with Broccoli on Cauliflower Rice

Preparation time: 5 minutes

Cooking time: 15 minutes

Servings: 2

Ingredients:

- 1 lb. of raw beef round steak, cut into strips.
- 1 tbsp. + 2 tsp. of low sodium soy sauce
- 1 Splenda packet
- ½ cup of water
- 1 ½ cup of broccoli florets
- 1 tsp. of sesame or olive oil
- 2 cups of cooked, grated cauliflower or frozen diced cauliflower

Directions:

1. Stir steak with soy and allow to sit for about 15 minutes.
2. Heat oil over medium-high heat and fry beef for 3-5 minutes or until browned.

3. Remove from pan.
4. Put broccoli, Splenda, and water in the pan. Cook for 5 minutes or until broccoli starts to appear soft, stirring sometimes.
5. Add beef back in and heat up thoroughly.
6. Serve the dish with cauliflower rice.

Nutrition:

- Calories 201
- Protein: 23 g
- Fat: 4 g
- Carbs: 2 g

Ancho Tilapia on Cauliflower Rice

Preparation time: 15 minutes

Cooking time: 30 minutes

Servings: 4

Ingredients:

- 2 lbs. of tilapia
- 1 tsp. of lime juice
- 1 tsp. of salt
- 1 tbsp. of ground ancho pepper
- 1 tsp. of ground cumin
- 1 ½ tbsp. of extra virgin olive oil
- ¼ cup of toasted pumpkin seeds
- 6 cups of cauliflower rice minutes
- 1 cup of coarsely chopped fresh cilantro

Directions:

1. Preheat oven to 450°F.
2. Dress tilapia with juice and put aside.

3. Combine cumin, ancho pepper, and salt in a bowl. Season tilapia with spice mixture.

4. Lay tilapia on a baking sheet or casserole dish and bake for 7 minutes.

5. In the meantime, in a big skillet, boil the cauliflower rice in olive oil till it becomes soft or for about 2-3 minutes.

6. Blend the pumpkin seeds and cilantro into the rice. Remove from heat, and serve.

Nutrition:

- Calories: 350
- Fat: 13 g
- Carbohydrate: 10 g
- Protein: 51 g

Turkey Caprese Meatloaf Cups

Preparation time: 20 minutes

Cooking time: 45 minutes

Servings: 6

Ingredients:

- 1 large egg
- 2 pounds of ground turkey breast
- 3 pieces of sun-dried tomatoes, drained and chopped
- ¼ cup of fresh basil leaves, chopped
- 5 ounces of low-fat fresh mozzarella; shredded
- ½ teaspoon of garlic powder
- ¼ teaspoon of salt and ½ teaspoon of pepper, to taste

Directions:

1. Preheat oven to 400°F.
2. Beat the egg in a big bowl.
3. Add the remaining Ingredients and blend everything with your hands until they are evenly combined.
4. Spray a 12-cup muffin tin and divide the turkey mixture among the muffin cups, pressing the combination in.

Cook in the preheated oven till the turkey is well-cooked or for about 25-30 minutes.

5. Chill the meatloaves entirely and store them in a container in the fridge for up to five days.

Nutrition:

- Calories: 181
- Protein: 43 g
- Fat: 11 g
- Carbs: 9 g

Almond Pancakes

Preparation time: 10 minutes

Cooking time: 13 minutes

Servings: 12

Ingredients:

- 6 eggs
- 1/4 cup of almonds; toasted
- 2 ounces of cocoa chocolate
- 1 teaspoon of almond extract
- 1/3 cup of coconut; shredded
- 1/2 teaspoon of baking powder
- 1/4 cup of coconut oil
- 1/2 cup of coconut flour
- 1/4 cup of stevia
- 1 cup of almond milk
- Cooking spray
- A pinch of salt

Directions:

1. Mix coconut flour with stevia, baking powder, salt, coconut, and stir.
2. Add coconut oil, eggs, almond milk and the flavorer and stir well again.
3. Add chocolate and almonds and whisk well again.
4. Heat up a pan and add cooking spray; add 2 tablespoons of batter, spread into a circle, cook until its golden, flip, cook again until it's done and transfer to a pan.
5. Do the same for rest of the batter and serve your pancakes directly.

Nutrition:

- Calories: 266
- Fat: 13 g
- Fiber: 8 g
- Carbs: 10 g
- Protein: 11 g

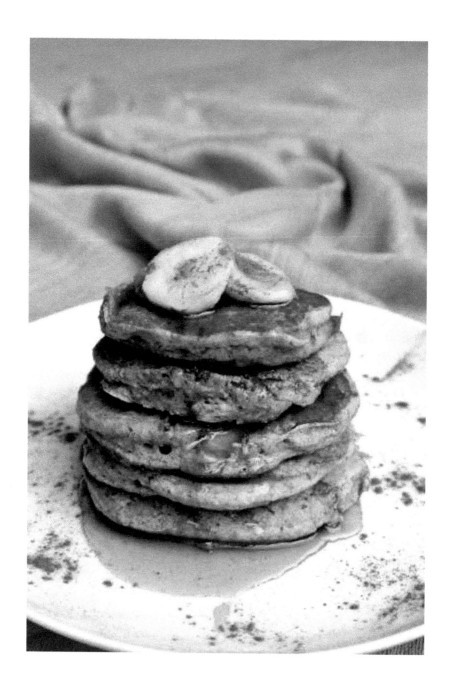